GUT HEALTH SMOOTHIE RECIPES BOOK

Delicious And Nutritious Recipes for Optimal Gut Health

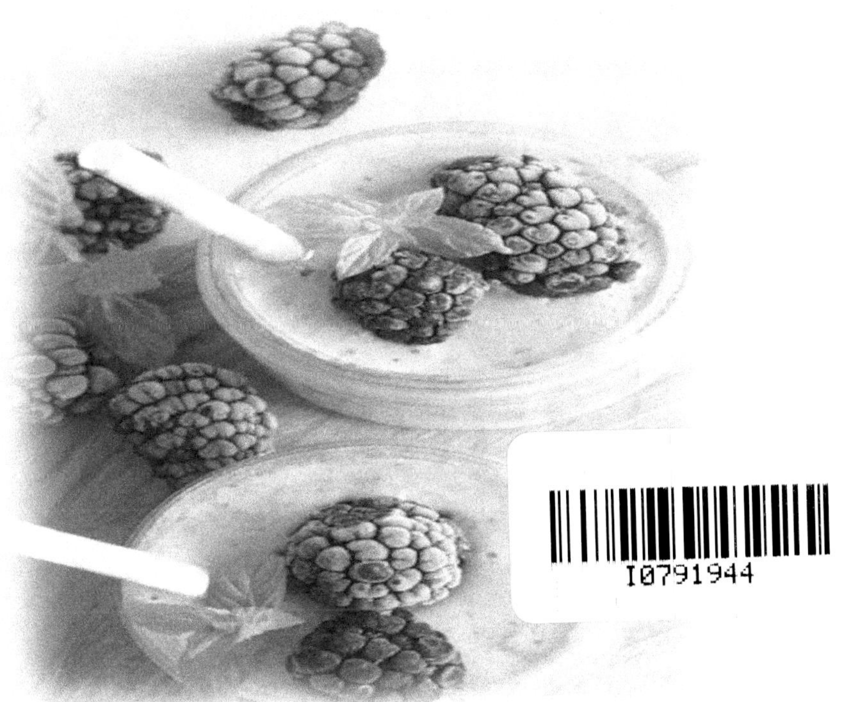

CHRISTIANA WHITE

GAIN ACCESS TO MORE BOOKS

TABLE OF CONTENTS.

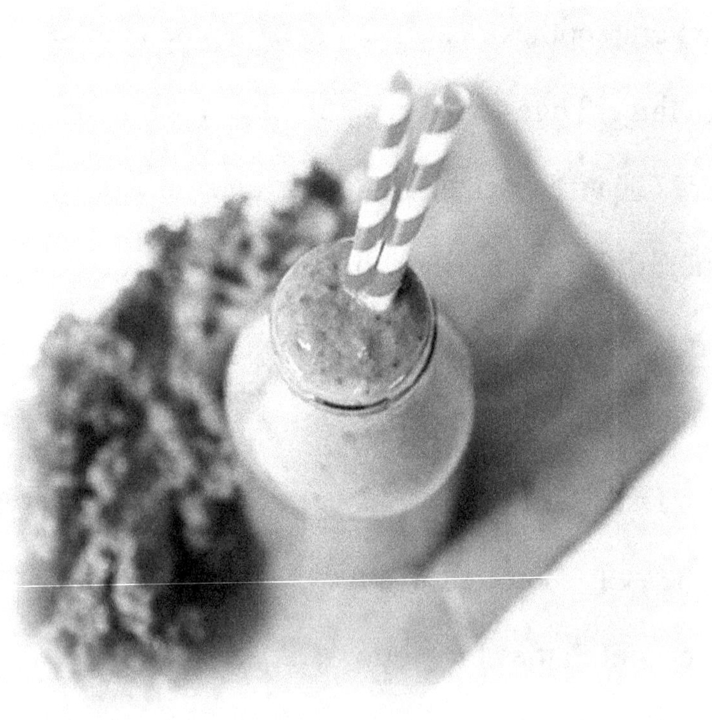

INTRODUCTION

Begin a revolutionary path to vitality with "The Gut Health Smoothie Recipes Book." This guide is more than just a compilation of recipes; it's a lifeline for individuals suffering from digestive issues. It serves as a monument to the power of natural healing, providing comfort and strength to those in need.

Consider a life free of the shackles of digestive discomfort, where each day is greeted without the fear of stomach pain. This goal has become a reality for many people because to the restorative properties of these expertly produced smoothies. Each formula is a combination of nature's best, intended to soothe, nourish, and revitalize your digestive system.

The pages of this book are packed with inspiring stories of change—stories of people who have made these smoothies a part of their daily routine, finding not only relief but joy in every cup. These blends are a symphony of flavor and health, with each component chosen for its capacity to promote digestive balance.

This book gives an open invitation to everybody who wants to enhance their gut health. Whether you want to relieve symptoms, boost your immune system, or simply enjoy delicious, wholesome beverages, this book will help you become a better, more vibrant version of yourself.

We sincerely thank you, the reader, for joining us on this wellness journey. Your drive to improved health is remarkable, and we are honoured to accompany you on this journey. As you read through these pages, take comfort in knowing that each recipe is good for not only your gut but also your entire health and happiness.

Join us on a journey of digestive wellness and vitality. Let the path to a healthier gut begin.

CHAPTER 1: UNDERSTANDING GUT HEALTH.

What is Gut Health?

Gut health refers to the overall health of our gastrointestinal system, which includes the stomach, small intestine, and large intestine. It is a sophisticated ecosystem with trillions of creatures, including bacteria.

These microorganisms have an important function in digestion, food absorption, and overall health. When our gut is healthy and thriving, it benefits our entire body.

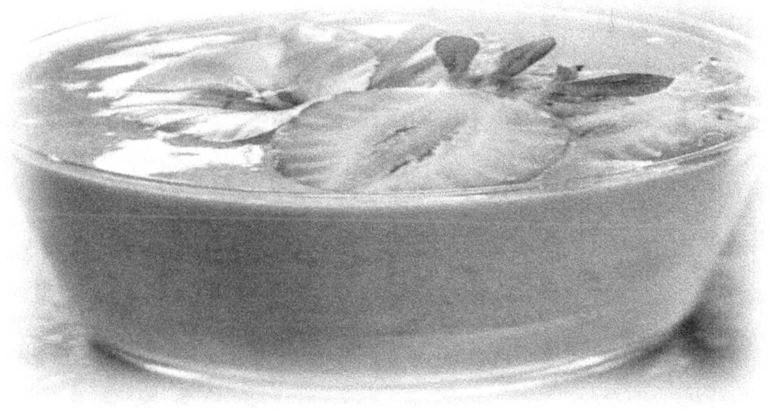

Importance of Gut Health

Maintaining a healthy gut is important for various reasons.

- Proper gut function leads to efficient digestion and nutrition absorption. It digests food, extracts vitamins, minerals, and energy, and transports them to the cells.

- Gut plays a significant role in immune system support, accounting for approximately 70%. A healthy gut regulates immune responses, thereby preventing infections and autoimmune diseases.

- Mental Health: The gut-brain connection is genuine. A healthy gut promotes mental well-being by lowering the risk of anxiety, depression, and cognitive decline.

- Weight Management: Gut bacteria affect metabolism and fat accumulation. An unbalanced stomach can cause weight gain or trouble decreasing weight.

- Controlling Inflammation: Chronic inflammation can lead to a variety of disorders. A healthy stomach reduces inflammation and promotes overall health.

Smoothies Have Gut Health Benefits.

Smoothies are an excellent way to nourish your gut. Here's why.

- Smoothies are a convenient way to eat a variety of nutrients due to their combination of gut-friendly ingredients. Think about leafy greens, fruits, and probiotic-rich foods.
- **Fiber Boost:** Fiber feeds healthy gut bacteria. Add chia seeds, flaxseeds, or oats to your smoothies for a fiber boost.
- **Probiotics**: Kefir, yogurt, and other fermented foods boost gut health by introducing helpful microorganisms. Include them in your smoothies.

- **Hydration**: Smoothies typically include water-rich fruits like watermelon and berries. Proper hydration improves intestinal function.

- **Antioxidants**: Berries, spinach, and other smoothie components include antioxidants that help protect gastrointestinal cells from harm.

Remember that sustaining intestinal health requires a broad diet rich in colorful, complete foods. So, blend up some gut-friendly smoothies and reap the advantages!

CHAPTER 2

Ingredients for Gut Health

Probiotics and prebiotics.

Probiotics are living bacteria that offer health advantages when eaten. They are sometimes referred to as 'good' or 'friendly' bacteria.

They help to maintain the gut flora, which is essential for digestion, immunological function, and overall health. Probiotic foods include yogurt, kefir, sauerkraut, tempeh, and kimchi.

Prebiotics are dietary fibres that feed the beneficial microorganisms in your stomach. This helps the gut bacteria create nutrients for your colon cells, resulting in a healthy digestive tract. Prebiotic-rich foods include garlic, onions, leeks, asparagus, bananas, and oats.

Fiber-Rich Fruits and Vegetables.

Fiber is necessary for a functioning digestive system. It helps you stay regular and promotes a healthy gut microbiota. Fruits and vegetables have high levels of soluble and insoluble fiber.

Soluble fiber dissolves in water and has been shown to reduce blood glucose and cholesterol levels. Apples, oranges, and strawberries, as well as carrots and psyllium husk, are high in soluble fiber.

Insoluble fiber does not dissolve in water and aids food passage through your digestive tract, supporting regularity. Dark leafy greens, root vegetable skins, fruit skins, and whole wheat products are good sources of insoluble fiber.

By including these ingredients into your smoothies, you'll be generating tasty, nutrient-dense beverages that can benefit your gut health and general well-being.

CHAPTER 3: SMOOTHIE BASICS

Equipment Required

To create tasty and healthy smoothies, you will need the following equipment:

- **Blenders**: A high-quality blender is required. Vitamix, Ninja, and Nutri bullet are popular options.

- **Ice Crusher**: For smoothies that require ice, an ice crusher or a blender with ice crushing capabilities is necessary.

- **Juicers**: If you want to add fresh juice to your smoothies, a decent juicer can be useful.

- **Knives and Cutting Boards:** Use sharp knives and sturdy cutting boards to prepare fruits and vegetables.

- **Measuring cups and scales:** Used to correctly measure substances.

- **Storage Containers**: Use Mason jars or large jugs to store smoothies in the refrigerator or freezer.

Tips For the Perfect Smoothie.

- Ingredient Order: Begin by combining leafy greens with liquid, then add remaining ingredients to achieve a smooth texture.

- Consistency: Use frozen fruits to keep your smoothie chilly and thick. If your smoothie is too thick, add extra liquid.

- Sweetness: If desired, add natural sweeteners such as honey, maple syrup, or Medjool dates.

- Blending: Begin with a low speed and gradually increase to high to get a homogeneous texture.

How To Store and Prepare Ingredients

- Refrigeration: Chill smoothies in airtight containers such as mason jars for 1-2 days.

- Freezing: Store smoothies or ingredients in freezer-safe containers for up to three months.

- Prep Packs: Make smoothie packs with all ingredients and freeze them. Blend until ready to drink.

- Dry Ingredients: Keep dry ingredients like oats and protein powder in sealed containers at room temperature.

By following these guidelines, you'll be well on your way to making gut-healthy smoothies that are both nutritious and tasty. Enjoy playing with different combinations and Flavors!

CHAPTER 4

Gut-Healing Smoothie Recipes

Classic Berry Probiotic Smoothie.

- ***Servings: Two.***
- ***Prep time: 5 minutes.***

Ingredients:

- 1 cup mixed berries, fresh or frozen.
- One cup of probiotic yogurt.
- One tablespoon of honey (optional)
- Half-cup water or almond milk

Instructions:

- Place the mixed berries and probiotic yogurt in a blender.
- If you want it sweeter, add honey.
- Add water or almond milk to reach the desired consistency.
- Blend until smooth.

- Serve immediately and enjoy!

Green Detox Smoothie

- *Serves: 1*
- *Prep time: 5 minutes.*

Ingredients:

- One cup spinach leaf.
- 1/2 green apple, sliced
- 1/2 cup chopped cucumber.
- One spoonful of chia seeds.
- One cup of coconut water.

Instructions:

- Add the spinach, green apple, and cucumber to the blender.
- Sprinkle with chia seeds.
- Pour the coconut water over the ingredients.
- Blend until smooth and completely incorporated.
- Savor this cleansing blend!

Golden Turmeric Smoothie

- ***Servings: Two.***
- ***Prep time: 5 minutes.***

Ingredients:

- One banana.
- 1 cup of pineapple pieces.
- 1/2 teaspoon of turmeric powder.
- 1/2 teaspoon grated ginger.
- One cup of almond milk.

Instructions:

- Place the banana and pineapple chunks in the blender.
- Combine turmeric powder and grated ginger.
- Add in the almond milk.
- Blend until you have a smooth, golden consistency.
- Serve this anti-inflammatory powerhouse!

Sweet Potato Ginger Smoothie

Ingredients:

- Two thumb-sized pieces of ginger, peeled
- 1/2 cup baked sweet potato.
- ¼ ripe avocado
- 1-2 soft dates, pitted
- 1 tablespoon cocoa powder.
- ¼ teaspoon cinnamon.
- 1/2 teaspoon Vanilla Extract.
- 1 cup of non-dairy milk, or more as needed.
- A sprinkling of nutmeg for garnish (optional).

Instructions:

- Combine all ingredients in a blender.
- If your blender isn't powerful enough, grate the ginger first.
- Blend at high speed until smooth and serve.

Beetroot and Berry Fiber Blast

Ingredients:

- 1/3 cup peeled and diced raw beet.

- 1 ⅓ cups frozen strawberries

- 1/4 ripe frozen banana (optional).

- 2/3 cup fresh apple juice.

- Garnish with fresh mint or shredded coconut (optional).

Instructions:

- Place the beet, strawberries, banana (if using), and apple juice in a blender.
- Blend on high until creamy and smooth, scraping down the sides as necessary.
- Taste and adjust the flavor as needed.

Creamy Avocado and Coconut Smoothie

Ingredients:

- Eight ice cubes.
- One medium avocado, diced.
- 1/2 cup low-fat vanilla yogurt.
- 1/2 cup whole milk.
- 1/4 cup cream of coconut.

Instructions:

- In a blender, combine ice cubes, avocado, yogurt, milk, and cream of coconut.
- Blend until smooth.

Pineapple Basil Digestives

- ***Servings: Two.***
- ***Prep time: 5 minutes.***

Ingredients:

- One cup of frozen pineapple pieces.
- One cup of coconut water.

- One-quarter cup basil leaves

- 1 teaspoon of agave syrup (or to taste).

- Three ice cubes.

Instructions:

- Place all items in a blender.

- Blend until smooth.

- Taste for sweetness and adjust as needed.

- Serve immediately.

Carrot Cake Prebiotic Smoothie.

- *Servings: Two.*

- *Prep time: 5 minutes.*

Ingredients:

- One huge ripe frozen banana.

- One small carrot, diced

- One pitted date (optional).

- 1/4 teaspoon ground cinnamon.

- 1/2 teaspoon vanilla extract.

- 1 tablespoon freshly chopped or grated ginger

- One generous pinch of ground nutmeg
- 1/2 - 1 cup dairy-free milk (use less for thicker smoothies and more for thinner smoothies).

Instructions:

- Combine banana, carrot, date (if using), cinnamon, vanilla, ginger, nutmeg, and dairy-free milk in a high-speed blender.
- Blend until creamy and smooth.
- Add more dairy-free milk as required to thicken or mix.

Kiwi Cucumber Refresher.

- *Serves: 1*
- *Prep time: 7 minutes.*

Ingredients:

- Two Kiwis.
- 1 cup chopped cucumber.
- 1/2 cup almond milk.
- Ice

Instructions:

- Peel and cut the kiwi into slices.

- Dice the cucumber until you have one cup.

- Place the kiwi, cucumber, almond milk, and a handful of ice in the blender.

- Blend until smooth.

Spicy Ginger Kombucha Zing.

- ***Servings vary.***
- ***Preparation Time: Varies***

Ingredients:

- Kombucha from the first fermentation.

- Fresh ginger (to taste)

- Hot pepper (e.g., jalapeno, chili, or habanero), optional

- Sugar (a combination of honey and brown sugar is ideal).

Instructions:

- Puree the ginger and sugar together.

- Transfer kombucha to fermentation bottles, evenly distributing the ginger combination and finishing with a few slices of pepper, if preferred.

- Ferment for 3 to 10 days, or until the desired carbonation level is achieved.

- Remove the ginger fibres and peppers (optional), and chill in the refrigerator before serving.

Please modify the amount of ginger and pepper to your liking for the Spicy Ginger Kombucha Zing, and be sure to use safe fermentation techniques.

Chocolate Banana Gut Comfort

- ***Servings: Two.***
- ***Prep time: 5 minutes.***

Ingredients:

- Two ripe bananas.
- One cup unsweetened almond milk.

- Two teaspoons of raw cacao powder.

- One spoonful of chia seeds.

- One teaspoon of pure vanilla extract.

- Ice cubes (Optional)

Instructions:

- Peel the bananas and put them into a blender.

- Combine almond milk, cacao powder, chia seeds, and vanilla extract.

- Blend on high until smooth. If you prefer a cooler consistency, add some ice cubes.

- Pour into glasses and serve immediately for the finest flavor and gut-healing effects.

Tangy Orange and Papaya Smoothie

- ***Servings: Two.***
- ***Prep time: 7 minutes.***

Ingredients:

- 1 cup fresh papaya, diced
- Juice from two big oranges

- One tablespoon of freshly grated ginger.

- One teaspoon of turmeric powder.

- One tablespoon of honey (optional)

- Ice cubes (Optional)

Instructions:

- In a blender, combine papaya, orange juice, ginger, and turmeric powder.

- Blend until smooth. If desired, add honey for sweetness.

- Add ice cubes to make a cold smoothie.

- Serve immediately, topped with a slice of orange or papaya, if desired.

<u>*Minty Melon Morning.*</u>

- ***Servings: Two.***
- ***Prep time: 5 minutes.***

Ingredients:

- 2 cups cubed honeydew melon.
- 1/2 cup of fresh mint leaves.
- One cup of coconut water.
- One tablespoon of lime juice.
- One teaspoon of spirulina powder (optional)

Instructions:

- Place the honeydew melon, mint leaves, coconut water, and lime juice in a blender.
- Blend until smooth. Spirulina powder can be added to provide an additional health boost.
- Serve chilled as a refreshing start to the day.

Almond Butter and Jelly

- *Serves: 1*
- *Prep time: 5 minutes.*

Ingredients:

- One cup unsweetened almond milk.
- Two tablespoons of almond butter.
- One-half cup frozen strawberries
- One spoonful of flaxseed meal.
- One teaspoon of honey (optional)

Instructions:

- In a blender, combine almond milk, almond butter, frozen strawberries, and flax seed meal.
- Blend until creamy. If desired, add honey for sweetness.
- Savor this nostalgic yet healthful smoothie.

<u>*Soothing Licorice Root Elixir*</u>

- ***Serves: 1***

- ***Prep Time: 5 minutes, including steeping time.***

Ingredients:

- One cup of boiling water.

- One teaspoon of licoricey root powder.

- One-half banana.

- One tablespoon of oats

- One teaspoon of honey (optional)

Instructions:

- Steep licoricey root powder in boiling water for 10 minutes, then cool.

- In a blender, mix the licoricey tea, banana, oats, and honey.

- Blend until smooth, then enjoy this calming beverage.

Pomegranate Punch Probiotic Power

- *Servings: Two.*
- *Prep time: 5 minutes.*

Ingredients:

- One cup of pomegranate seeds
- 1 cup kefir or probiotic yogurt.
- One banana.
- One tablespoon of honey (optional)

Instructions:

- Combine pomegranate seeds, kefir, and banana in a blender.
- Blend until smooth. Adjust sweetness with honey to taste.
- Serve immediately to preserve the probiotic benefits.

<u>*Lemon Ginger Zest Cleanse.*</u>

- ***Serves: 1***
- ***Prep time: 5 minutes.***

Ingredients:

- One cup of filtered water.
- Juice from one large lemon.
- One tablespoon of freshly grated ginger.
- One teaspoon of apple cider vinegar.
- 1/2 teaspoon of ground turmeric.
- One teaspoon of honey (optional)

Instructions:

- Mix water, lemon juice, ginger, apple cider vinegar, and turmeric in a blender.
- Blend until well combined. If desired, add honey for sweetness.
- Drink this zesty smoothie first thing in the morning to jumpstart your digestive system.

Savory Tomato Smoothie.

- **_Servings: Two._**
- **_Prep time: 10 minutes._**

Ingredients:

- 2 cups ripe tomatoes, chopped
- One-half cup carrot juice
- 1/4 cup chopped celery.
- One tablespoon of lemon juice.
- One-half teaspoon sea salt
- One sprinkle of cayenne pepper (optional)

Instructions:

- Add tomatoes, carrot juice, celery, and lemon juice to a blender.
- Blend until smooth. Season with sea salt and cayenne pepper.
- Serve chilled for a flavorful, gastrointestinal-friendly treat.

Watermelon Mint Hydration

- ***Servings: Two.***

- ***Prep time: 5 minutes.***

Ingredients:

- Four cups of diced watermelon

- 1/4 cup of fresh mint leaves.

- Juice from 1 lime

- One cup of coconut water.

Instructions:

- Combine watermelon, mint leaves, lime juice, and coconut water in a blender.

- Blend until smooth and frothy.

- Pour into glasses and serve immediately for a refreshing hydration boost.

Apple Cinnamon Fiber-Rich

- ***Servings: Two.***
- ***Prep time: 5 minutes.***

Ingredients:

- Two apples, cored and sliced
- One cup unsweetened almond milk.
- 1/2 teaspoon of ground cinnamon.
- One tablespoon of ground flaxseed
- One teaspoon of honey (optional)

Instructions:

- In a blender, combine apples, almond milk, cinnamon, and flax seeds.
- Blend until smooth. If desired, add honey for sweetness.
- Top with a sprinkling of cinnamon for a fiber-rich, gut-healthy smoothie.

<u>*Tropical Mango Tango*</u>

- ***Servings: Two.***
- ***Prep time: 5 minutes.***

Ingredients:

- One ripe mango, peeled and diced
- 1 cup of pineapple pieces.
- One banana.
- One cup of coconut milk.
- One tablespoon of lime juice.
- Ice cubes (Optional)

Instructions:

- Blend mango, pineapple, banana, coconut milk, and lime juice.
- Blend until smooth. If you prefer a cooler consistency, add some ice cubes.
- Serve immediately for a tropical gut-health boost.

<u>*Berry Spinach Boost*</u>

- ***Servings: Two.***
- ***Prep time: 5 minutes.***

Ingredients:

- 1 cup mixed berries (strawberries, raspberries, blueberries)
- 1 cup fresh spinach leaves.
- One banana.
- One cup of almond milk.
- One spoonful of chia seeds.

Instructions:

- Put the berries, spinach, banana, almond milk, and chia seeds in a blender.
- Blend until smooth and creamy.
- This antioxidant-rich smoothie can be enjoyed at any time.

<u>*Chia Seed Omega Mix.*</u>

- *Serves: 1*
- *Prep time: 5 minutes.*

Ingredients:

- One cup unsweetened almond milk.
- Two teaspoons of chia seeds.
- One-half banana.
- One-quarter cup blueberries
- One teaspoon of honey (optional)

Instructions:

- Soak the chia seeds in almond milk for 20 minutes until they become gelatinous.
- Combine soaked chia seeds, banana, and blueberries in a blender.
- Blend until smooth. If desired, add honey for sweetness.
- Drink this smoothie high in omega-3 fatty acids to improve intestinal health.

<u>*Red Velvet Healing Smoothie.*</u>

- ***Servings: Two.***
- ***Prep time: 5 minutes.***

Ingredients:

- 1/2 cup cooked beets, peeled and chopped
- One cup unsweetened almond milk.
- One-half ripe avocado
- Two teaspoons of raw cacao powder.
- One tablespoon of honey (optional)

Instructions:

- Blend beets, almond milk, avocado, and cacao powder.
- Blend until smooth. If desired, add honey for sweetness.
- Serve this nutrient-dense smoothie as a tasty gut health treat.

<u>*Pumpkin Spice Probiotic*</u>

- ***Servings: Two.***
- ***Prep time: 5 minutes.***

Ingredients:

- 1/2 cup pumpkin puree.
- 1 cup kefir or probiotic yogurt.
- One banana.
- 1/2 teaspoon of pumpkin spice mix.
- 1 tablespoon of maple syrup (optional).

Instructions:

- Blend the pumpkin puree, kefir, banana, and pumpkin spice mix until smooth.
- Add maple syrup if desired.
- Drink this seasonal probiotic-rich smoothie for intestinal health.

Aloe Vera Soothes

- *Serves: 1*
- *Prep time: 5 minutes.*

Ingredients:

- One cup aloe vera juice.
- 1/2 cucumber, peeled and sliced.
- 1/2 cup fresh pineapple pieces.
- One tablespoon of honey (optional)

Instructions:

- Blend the aloe vera juice, cucumber, and pineapple until smooth.
- Add honey if desired.
- Drink this calming smoothie to relax your digestive system.

<u>*Pear Ginger Digestive Aid.*</u>

- ***Servings: Two.***
- ***Prep time: 5 minutes.***

Ingredients:

- Two ripe pears, cored and sliced
- One tablespoon of freshly grated ginger.
- 1 cup water or coconut water.
- One teaspoon of honey (optional)

Instructions:

- In a blender, combine pear, ginger, and water.
- Blend until smooth. If you want to sweeten it, add honey.
- Use this digestive-friendly smoothie for a light gut cleanse.

Celery Cleanse Cocktail

- ***Serves: 1***
- ***Prep time: 5 minutes.***

Ingredients:

- 4 stalks celery.
- One apple, cored and sliced
- One tablespoon of lemon juice.
- One cup of water.

Instructions:

- Juice the celery and apple, then transfer to a blender.
- Add lemon juice and water, then mix until smooth.
- Drink this cocktail for detoxifying and digestion.

<u>*Grapefruit Rosemary Remedy*</u>

- *Servings: Two.*
- *Prep time: 5 minutes.*

Ingredients:

- One grapefruit, peeled and seeded
- One fresh sprig of rosemary
- 1 cup water or coconut water.
- One teaspoon of honey (optional)

Instructions:

- Blend the grapefruit, rosemary, and water until smooth.
- Strain if desired, then sweeten with honey.
- This therapy is ideal for lowering inflammation and promoting intestinal health.

Cherry Almond Antioxidant

- *Servings: Two.*
- *Prep time: 5 minutes.*

Ingredients:

- One cup frozen cherry.
- One cup unsweetened almond milk.
- Two tablespoons of almond butter.
- One teaspoon of vanilla extract.

Instructions:

- In a blender, mix cherries, almond milk, almond butter, and vanilla essence.
- Blend until creamy.
- Drink this antioxidant-rich smoothie for a healthy stomach.

<u>*Blueberry Flaxseed Focus*</u>

- ***Servings: Two.***
- ***Prep time: 5 minutes.***

Ingredients:

- One cup blueberry.
- One cup unsweetened almond milk.
- Two teaspoons of ground flaxseed.
- One banana.

Instructions:

- Blend the blueberries, almond milk, flaxseed, and banana until smooth.
- Serve this omega-3-rich smoothie to promote brain and gastrointestinal health.

<u>*Cacao Date Recovery*</u>

- ***Serves: 1***
- ***Prep time: 5 minutes.***

Ingredients:

- Two teaspoons of raw cacao powder.
- Three pitted dates.
- One cup unsweetened almond milk.
- One banana.

Instructions:

- Soak the dates in almond milk for 10 minutes to soften.
- Place-soaked dates, cacao powder, and banana in a blender.
- Blend until smooth and serve as a post-workout recovery treat.

Raspberry Lemonade Laxative.

- ***Servings: Two.***
- ***Prep time: 5 minutes.***

Ingredients:

- One cup raspberry.
- Juice from 2 lemons
- One tablespoon of honey (optional)
- One cup of water.

Instructions:

- Puree the raspberries, lemon juice, and water until smooth.
- Add honey if desired.
- This smoothie is ideal for natural constipation cure.

Peppermint Patties Probiotic

- ***Serves: 1***
- ***Prep time: 5 minutes.***

Ingredients:

- One cup of probiotic yogurt.
- One tablespoon of cacao nibs.
- 1/4 teaspoon of peppermint extract.
- One teaspoon of honey (optional)

Instructions:

- Blend the yogurt, cacao nibs, and peppermint essence until smooth.
- Optional: sweeten with honey.
- Indulge in this delicious probiotic-rich smoothie.

Fig and Honey Harmony

- ***Servings: Two.***
- ***Prep time: 5 minutes.***

Ingredients:

- Six fresh figs, stemmed and halved.
- One cup of Greek yogurt.
- Two teaspoons of honey.
- 1/2 teaspoon of ground cinnamon.

Instructions:

- Blend the figs, yogurt, honey, and cinnamon until smooth.
- Serve this fiber-rich smoothie to promote intestinal harmony.

<u>*Citrus Immune Boosters*</u>

- ***Servings: Two.***
- ***Prep time: 5 minutes.***

Ingredients:

- Juice from 2 oranges
- Juice from 1 grapefruit
- One tablespoon of grated ginger.
- One teaspoon of turmeric powder.
- One tablespoon of honey (optional)

Instructions:

- In a blender, combine the citrus juice, ginger, and turmeric.
- Blend until well combined. If desired, add honey for sweetness.
- Drink this immune-boosting smoothie to improve gut health.

<u>*Avocado-Mint Digestive Aid*</u>

- ***Servings: Two.***
- ***Prep time: 5 minutes.***

Ingredients:

- One ripe avocado.
- One cup spinach leaf.
- 1/4 cup of fresh mint leaves.
- One tablespoon of lemon juice.
- One cup of coconut water.
- One teaspoon of honey (optional)

Instructions:

- Scoop out the avocado flesh and transfer it to a blender.
- Combine the spinach, mint leaves, lemon juice, and coconut water.
- Blend until smooth. If desired, add honey for sweetness.
- Drink this creamy smoothie to ease digestion.

<u>*Papaya Pineapple Enzyme Booster*</u>

- ***Servings: Two.***
- ***Prep time: 5 minutes.***

Ingredients:

- 1 cup fresh papaya, diced
- 1 cup fresh pineapple, diced
- One banana.
- One cup of coconut milk.
- One tablespoon of lime juice.

Instructions:

- In a blender, mix papaya, pineapple, banana, coconut milk, and lime juice.
- Blend until smooth.
- Serve this enzyme-rich smoothie to promote digestive health.

<u>*Spicy Tomato Cleanser*</u>

- ***Servings: Two.***
- ***Prep time: 5 minutes.***

Ingredients:

- 2 cups ripe tomatoes, chopped
- One-quarter cup carrot juice
- 1/4 cup chopped celery.
- One tablespoon of lemon juice.
- 1/2 teaspoon of cayenne pepper.
- One pinch of sea salt.

Instructions:

- Add tomatoes, carrot juice, celery, lemon juice, cayenne pepper, and sea salt to a blender.
- Blend until smooth.
- Drink this spicy smoothie to cleanse and replenish your intestines.

Chocolate Almond Prebiotic Shake.

- ***Servings: Two.***
- ***Prep time: 5 minutes.***

Ingredients:

- Two cups of unsweetened almond milk.
- Two tablespoons of almond butter.
- Two teaspoons of raw cacao powder.
- One banana.
- 1 tablespoon of agave syrup or honey (optional).

Instructions:

- In a blender, mix almond milk, almond butter, cacao powder, and banana.
- Blend until creamy. Sweeten with agave syrup or honey if desired.
- Serve this prebiotic-rich shake to support your gut flora.

CONCLUSION

In composing the concluding words of our journey through the rich landscape of gut health smoothies, we go deeper into the substance of this book, intending to leave you with a lasting impression and a clear road forward.

Our investigation has uncovered the transforming power of gut health smoothies. Each formula is a tapestry weaved with the threads of nutritional science, meant to boost your digestive system.

The probiotics, prebiotics, fiber, and healthy fats that dance through these pages are more than ordinary ingredients; they are the architects of well-being, establishing a resilient gut microbiome that stands as the cornerstone of your health.

The route to wellness is not a sprint but a marathon, with each smoothie acting as both sustenance and motivation along the way. As you turn the blender on, let it symbolize the start of another day committed to your well-being. Let the whir of the blades be a reminder that you are taking active steps toward a healthier, happier self.

This book is a companion, a guide to join you on your wellness journey. However, it is not a solo route. The wisdom of healthcare specialists is a great asset, illuminating the road ahead with individualized guidance tailored to your particular health narrative.

Their knowledge guarantees that the journey you embark upon not only leads to greater health but is performed with the highest care and regard for your unique needs.

If the pages of this book have enhanced your life, if the smoothies have brought a new zest to your days, I sincerely ask that you share your experiences. Your favorable comment is not simply a kind gesture; it's a beacon for others navigating the enormous sea of health information. It's a statement that the recipes within these pages are more than just a collection of ingredients; they are a catalyst for change.

As we part ways, remember that this book is not a conclusion but a beginning. A beginning of a more mindful, health-focused approach to living. A beginning of a connection with food that is as soothing as it is delightful.

And most crucially, a beginning of a new chapter in your life, one where you stand at the helm, steering yourself toward a horizon of vigorous health and energy.

May your blender always be full, and your journey always be fruitful.